MW01248144

Cytotec Misoprostol

The Ultimate Guide to Use the Abortion Pill during the Early Part of Pregnancy

Jacob Ryan

Title | CYTOTEC MISOPROSTOL
Author | Jacob Ryan
ISBN | 979-12-22751-37-5

Youcanprint
Via Marco Biagi 6, 73100 Lecce
www.youcanprint.it
info@youcanprint.it
Made by human

Chapter 1: What You Should Know about Cytotec

What is Cytotec (Misoprostol)?

Cytotec, or misoprostol as it is more often known, is a pros-taglandin. It functions similarly to the prostaglandins that are naturally created by your organism. Prostaglandins are molecules that support preserving the belly from harm and ulcerations. Not only can nonsteroidal anti-inflammatory drugs (NSAIDs) reduce the number of prostaglandins found in the stomach region, but the medicine itself can injure the stomach. Because of this, some patients who take NSAIDs may also be given the prescription medication misoprostol (Cytotec), which lowers the chance of developing stomach ulcers.

Misoprostol stimulates the uterus to contract and empty, which is beneficial for women who are undergoing a medical abortion or who are attempting to induce labor with the medicine.

The following is a list of the two diastereomers that are found in about equal concentrations in misoprostol, along with their respective enantiomers denoted by the symbol ($\pm$):

What is Mifepristone (RU-486)?

When terminating a pregnancy that has lasted less than seventy days, a combination of the medications mifepristone and miso-prostol is typically utilized. It accomplishes this by interrupting the flow of hormones that are responsible for keeping the uterine lining healthy. The uterus is unable to maintain the pregnancy in the absence of these hormones, and as a result, the contents of the uterus are ejected.

Mifepristone is also employed in the treatment of hyperglycemia, which refers to elevated blood sugar levels, in individuals with Cushing's syndrome who also suffer from type 2 diabetes and for whom surgery has been unsuccessful or who are not candidates for the procedure.

You need to have a medical recipe for this drug with the aim of purchasing it. It can only be procured from your medical practi-tioner. With the purchase of this medication, you have the option of purchasing the following dosage forms:

- Tablet

Properties and Characteristics of Cytotec

Experimental Properties

PROPERTY	VALUE
melting point	261-263

(°C)	
water solubility	1.6mg/mL

Predicted Properties

PROPERTY	VALUE
Water Solubility	0.0164 mg/mL
logP	3.88
logP	3.86
logS	-4.4
pKa (Strongest Acidic)	14.69
pKa (Strongest Basic)	-0.95
Physiological Charge	0
Hydrogen Acceptor Count	4
Hydrogen Donor Count	2
Polar Surface Area	83.83 Å^2
Rotatable Bond Count	14

Refractivity	107.88 $m^3 \cdot mol^{-1}$
Polarizability	45.44 $\mathring{A}^3$
Number of Rings	1
Bioavailability	1
Rule of Five	Yes
Ghose Filter	Yes
Veber's Rule	No
MDDR-like Rule	No

Predicted ADMET Features

PROPERTY	VALUE	PROBABILITY
Human Intestinal Absorption	+	0.9157
Blood Brain Barrier	+	0.938
Caco-2 permeable	-	0.5339
P-glycoprotein substrate	Substrate	0.6607
P-glycoprotein inhibitor I	Non-inhibitor	0.7261
P-glycoprotein inhibitor II	Inhibitor	0.6504
Renal organic	Non-inhibitor	0.9146

cation transporter		
CYP450 2C9 substrate	Non-substrate	0.857
CYP450 2D6 substrate	Non-substrate	0.9024
CYP450 3A4 substrate	Substrate	0.6281
CYP450 1A2 substrate	Non-inhibitor	0.8358
CYP450 2C9 inhibitor	Non-inhibitor	0.8175
CYP450 2D6 inhibitor	Non-inhibitor	0.9459
CYP450 2C19 inhibitor	Non-inhibitor	0.8199
CYP450 3A4 inhibitor	Non-inhibitor	0.795
CYP450 inhibitory promiscuity	Low CYP Inhibitory Promiscuity	0.9591
Ames test	Non AMES toxic	0.8289
Carcinogenicity	Non-carcinogens	0.8941
Biodegradation	Not ready biodegradable	0.8797
Rat acute toxicity	3.7051 LD50,	Not applicable

	mol/kg	
hERG inhibition (predictor I)	Weak inhibitor	0.964
hERG inhibition (predictor II)	Non-inhibitor	0.8734

History of Cytotec

Cytotec was first made available as a therapy for stomach and duodenal ulcers in the middle of the year 1986. 1992 was the year that saw sales reach their all-time low (150,207 vs. 189,199-581,003 annual sales). A newspaper campaign by anti-Cytotec organizations and a law that required a double-copy prescription were two other reasons that contributed to the decline in sales. The reduction in manufacturing was due to an agreement between the company and the MOH. Surveys conducted in hospitals in the early 1990s revealed that a significant number of women had taken Cytotec to bring on an abortion. The information that Cytotec may be used to induce an abortion was disseminated through the media, pharmacies, medical professionals, women, and the company. In order to induce an abortion, women often take 4-16 doses of Cytotec throughout the first trimester of their pregnancies. Cytotec is used because it may be administered discreetly, has a lower risk of side effects compared to other abortion procedures, and is reasonably affordable. Cytotec is thought to be risk-free by women as well. Despite this, the vast majority of pregnant women express dissatisfaction with the pain they endure and their ultimate need to seek medical attention. These unfavorable opinions are the result of a lack of knowledge regarding the actual mechanism by which the medicine is produced.

When to use Cytotec and Mifepristone?

These medication regimens are safe and effective. Ultrasonography or a woman's menstrual history can be used to estimate a woman's gestational age. When clinical data alone are not sufficient to confirm the gestational date of a pregnancy, or when there are risk factors for an ectopic pregnancy, ultrasonography is required. Mifepristone, which is a progesterone receptor antagonist, is taken orally in a dosage of 200 milligrams, and then misoprostol, which is a prostaglandin E1 analogue, is taken buccally or vaginally in a dosage of 800 milligrams. The drugs are known to cause cramping and bleeding as a side effect, with bleeding typically lasting between nine and sixteen days on average. The unwanted side effects of misoprostol, such as mild fever and gastrointestinal problems, are treatable with nonsteroidal anti-inflammatory medications (NSAIDs) or antiemetics. Rare problems include an ongoing pregnancy, an infection, bleeding, an undetected ectopic pregnancy, and the requirement for an unexpected uterine aspiration. It is possible to determine whether or not the pregnancy tissue has completely passed through the body by using clinical history in conjunction with serial quantitative beta human chorionic gonadotropin levels, urine pregnancy tests, or ultrasonography.

Chapter 2: How Does Cytotec Work?

Mechanism of Action of Cytotec

Misoprostol is a synthetic prostaglandin E1 analog that inhibits the production of gastric acid in the stomach by activating the prostaglandin E1 receptors that are found on the parietal cells of the stomach. This leads in less acid being created by the belly. This brings to a diminution in the volume of sourness that is produced in the belly. An increase in the production of mucus and bicarbonate, as well as a thickening of the mucosal bilayer, are necessary for the mucosa to be able to form new cells. This is accomplished by the mucosa thickening. All of this activity is carried out with the goal of getting the mucosa ready for the creation of new cells.

The ability of misoprostol to bind to smooth muscle cells in the uterine lining results in an increase in the intensity of the uterine contractions as well as an increase in the number of times they occur. It has the ability to break down collagen, and it can also reduce the tone in the cervix of the cervical cavity.

Mechanism of Action of Mifepristone

It is the intracellular receptors of the hormones that are antagonized that are involved in the mechanism of action (progesterone and glucocorticosteroids). All of these characteristics contribute to the binder's capacity to link to its objective. When contrasted with agonists, these particularities have ramifications at different stages of the receptor function. The logic, however, can't only be confined to the interaction that takes place between RU486 and the receptor. For example, there is the potential for a flip from an antagonistic property to an agonist activity, depending on the involvement of other signaling pathways in the process. If the line of reasoning was restricted to the interaction between RU486 and the receptor, then this would be the case. In spite of the similarities that exist between the structures of steroids, the receptors that are involved, and the response machinery in target cells, it would be advantageous to have derivatives with only one of the two antagonistic properties (antiprogestin, antiglucocorticosteroid).

Pharmacodynamics of Cytotec

Misoprostol, a prostaglandin E1 analog medication, reduces the risk of gastric ulcers caused by nonsteroidal anti-inflammatory medicines (NSAIDs) by preventing the generation of acid in the parietal cells of the stomach. In addition to its use in the treatment of miscarriages, misoprostol may also be utilized in the performance of first-trimester abortions, either on its own or in conjunction with mifepristone. When taken orally, a dosage of misoprostol begins to exert its effects around 8 minutes after administration, and these effects continue for roughly 2 hours. Misoprostol's beginning of action is delayed by approximately 8 minutes. When used sublingually, a single dose begins to exert its effects roughly 11 minutes after administration, and these effects continue for nearly three hours. The effect of a dosage that is administered vaginally begins to take effect after roughly 20 minutes and continues for around 4 hours. After one hundred minutes, a dose that is administered rectal will begin to exert its effects, which will last for a period of four hours.

Pharmacokinetics of Cytotec

The oral administration of Cytotec results in a quick absorption of the medication, with peak plasma levels of the active metabolite (misoprostol acid) arriving after around thirty minutes. Following repeated administration of a dose of 400 micrograms twice a day, there is no buildup of misoprostol acid in the plasma.

Combination of Cytotec and Mifepristone

Abortion by medical means, sometimes known as "medical abortion," is a non-surgical treatment in which medications are used to produce a spontaneous abortion. Mifepristone and misoprostol are the two drugs that are necessary for a medical abortion to be carried out in the most successful and risk-free manner. Mifepristone inhibits the action of progesterone, which in turn increases the uterine muscle's capacity to contract and initiates the embryo's separation from the uterine wall. The drug misoprostol causes the uterus to go into forceful contractions, which results in the expulsion of the products of conception. This process is pretty similar to that of an abortion that occurs naturally or a miscarriage. Induction of abortion can also be accomplished with the repeated injection of misoprostol alone. The cervix is made more pliable and the opening is made larger by both medicines.

Counseling, confirmation of intrauterine pregnancy, and estimation of the patient's gestational age should all be included in high-quality abortion care. Counseling on family planning and contraception should be offered either at the time of the abortion or after it has been performed. Abortion is now more readily available to women thanks to the development of medical abortion choices, which have also made it more acceptable for women to undergo medical abortions in the privacy and comfort of their own homes.

All of the methods include administering 200 milligrams of mifepristone followed by 800 micrograms of misoprostol through the vaginal canal, the buccal cavity, or the sublingual tract. For pregnancies with a gestational age of up to 9 weeks, the misoprostol dosage is given between 24 and 48 hours after the mifepristone dose. For pregnancies with a gestational age of 9 to 12 weeks and beyond 12 weeks, the misoprostol dose is taken between 36 and 48 hours after the mifepristone dose. It is possible that further misoprostol dosages of 400 mg will be necessary depending on the gestational age of the patient. More than ninety-five percent of women who follow these protocols have their pregnancies end in a successful abortion, and the risk of the pregnancy extending beyond 63 days after the last menstrual period is less than one percent.

The research that has been conducted to this point indicates that the complete abortion rates in early pregnancy with misoprostol-only regimens can range anywhere from 76% to 96%. Even though the regimen of mifepristone followed by misoprostol is much more effective than the use of misoprostol alone for early MA, misoprostol is typically more readily accessible than mifepristone, and it has been used alone for MA safely and successfully across the world. Misoprostol alone for early MA is significantly less effective than the use of misoprostol in combination with mifepristone. The combination of mifepristone and misoprostol is much more successful than either medication used on its own in the treatment of unwanted pregnancies. Both the World Health Organization (WHO) and the International Federation of Gynecology and Obstetrics (FIGO) suggest the administration of 800 mg of misoprostol vaginally or sublingually in pregnancies up to 12 weeks of gestation when mifepristone cannot be acquired. It is recommended that you carry out this treatment three times during the span of three to twelve hours. For pregnant women who are between 12 and 24 weeks of gestation, the prescribed quantity is lowered in half, and the prescription can be taken as often as five times every three hours.

Medical abortion has not been connected to any negative consequences on a patient's health in the long run, and it is statistically less harmful than maintaining a pregnancy. The utilization of the abortion medications mifepristone and misoprostol is very risk-free. Abortion by medicinal means may be more desirable than abortion through surgical means for certain women and the clinicians who care for them. Abortion by medical means is less invasive than abortion through surgical means, and hence, some women may have the impression that it is a more private process.

How to use them together?

Pregnancy's stage and the	First Day	Second Day

medicine being taken		
Mifepristone and misoprostol were used to terminate the pregnancy when the woman was less than 12 weeks pregnant.	Cytotec is designed to be ingested, with the first dosage beginning at 200 milligrams.	Approximately 24 hours after taking mifepristone, you should take 800 mcg of misoprostol, which is divided into four pills of 200 mcg each. You may do this by inserting two pills into each of your cheek pouches (the space between your teeth and your cheek), or you can place all four tablets beneath your tongue.
12 weeks pregnant or more, with the option to terminate the pregnancy using	Mifepristone is should be taken orally, with the first dose beginning at 200 mg.	About 24 hours after taking mifepristone, you should take 400 mcg of misoprostol, which is divided into two pills of 200 mcg each. You may do

mifepristone and misoprostol. this by inserting one tablet into each of your cheek pouches, or you can choose to place both tablets beneath your tongue at the same time. After three hours have elapsed, you will be required to take an additional dose of misoprostol equal to 400 mcg (two tablets of 200 mcg each). If you haven't had any cramping or bleeding yet, you should take another dosage of the same quantity of misoprostol three hours after the first one. This time, however, you should wait until after the first 3 hours have

	gone.	
Women who are less than 12 weeks pregnant and are just taking misoprostol	It is possible to consume 800 mcg of misoprostol, which is the same as taking four tablets that are each 200 mcg in strength. Either insert two pills in each of your cheek pouches (the space between your teeth and your cheek) or place all four tablets beneath your tongue in order to do this.	N/A
12 weeks pregnant or more, using just misoprostol to induce labor	You may administer dosages of misoprostol ranging from 50	N/A

mcg to 400 mcg by inserting one tablet into each of your cheek pouches or by placing both tablets under your tongue. Each cheek pouch should contain one tablet. Each pill contains a total of 200 mcg. After three hours have elapsed, you will be required to take an additional dose of misoprostol equal to 400 mcg (two tablets of 200 mcg each). If you haven't had any cramping or bleeding yet, you should take another dosage of

the same quantity

of misoprostol

three hours after

the first one. This

time, however,

you should wait

until after the first

3 hours have

gone.

What can you anticipate happening on day one?

Mifepristone is to be taken orally on day one, beginning with a dose of 200 milligrams (mg), which is equivalent to one tablet. It is possible that bleeding and other adverse effects will not manifest themselves for around twenty-four hours after taking mifepristone.

What can you anticipate happening on day 2?

If you are less than 12 weeks expectant, take 800 mcg (it is recommended to take misoprostol in the form of pills of 200 mcg each) roughly 24 hours after taking mifepristone. Either place all four pills beneath your tongue or place two tablets into each of your cheek pouches. This will ascertain that the medication is well absorbed. The use of misoprostol will result in the onset of labor and will terminate the pregnancy. You should take 800 mcg if you are pregnant for more than 12 weeks (two 400-mcg tablets).

After inserting one tablet of misoprostol into each cheek pouch or putting one tablet under the tongue and waiting thirty minutes, the next step is to drink a glass of water to flush out any traces of the drug that may still be present. Be secure to drink enough liquids throughout the day in order not to get dewatered.

Women who are 12 weeks pregnant or more should take 400 mcg (two tablets of 200 mcg each) of misoprostol approximately 24 hours after taking mifepristone. This can be done by adding one pill into each jowl, or by positioning both pills under the tongue. If you wish to terminate the pregnancy as soon as possible, you need to observe these steps.

After three hours have elapsed, you will be required to take an additional dose of misoprostol equal to 400 mcg (two tablets of 200 mcg each). If you haven't had any cramping or bleeding yet, you should take another dosage of the same quantity of misoprostol three hours after the first one. This time, however, you should wait until after the first 3 hours have gone.

The majority of the time, the beginning of unpleasant effects happens anywhere between 30 minutes to 10 hours after taking a misoprostol pill. At times, it may even take longer. When both of these medications are used, it may take anywhere from two to twenty-four hours for the body to rid itself of any traces of the pregnancy that may have been present.

How can one tell whether the pregnancy is no longer viable?

The earlier a medical abortion is carried out, the greater the likelihood that the embryo (which might appear as either gray or white tissue) would be absorbed by a blood clot without being detected. After it has been extracted, the cramping and bleeding should lessen.

Embryos do not reach a size greater than one inch in diameter until around nine weeks following the first day of the woman's most recent menstrual cycle.

What can you anticipate happening between days 3 and 5?

A "second wave" of significant bleeding is something that might happen a few days after you have successfully delivered the baby. Especially during the fourth and fifth day, you may have a rise in cramping, accompanied with bleeding and clotting.

It is possible that having someone touch your back, sitting on the toilet, or taking a shower can assist alleviate any discomfort; however, this will depend on how you are currently feeling.

If you are having significant bleeding, you should provide a gentle massage for around ten minutes on the regions of your abdomen, uterus, and pelvis. You might try taking acetaminophen or ibuprofen, applying a heating pad, and reducing the amount of additional physical activity you do as well.

If your fever stays at or above 101.4 degrees Fahrenheit (38.6 degrees Celsius) for more than 12 hours in a row, you may be facing a serious medical issue.

During this moment, you have the option to:

- Notice enormous blood clots, some as big as a lemon, in the patient.
- You may experience severe abdominal pain, diarrhea, mild fever or chills for a short period of time, mild to moderate nausea, and vomiting.
- Release a creamy substance from your nipple.

How to confirm that the abortion worked?

Make a note of the date as well as the result that you obtained, and then take another pregnancy test the week after that one.

If the outcomes of the first and second tests are both negative, it is quite likely that the abortion was successful as planned. If the results of both tests are identical, you don't have to act further.

Effectiveness of Cytotec

Women who had an anembryonic pregnancy had the lowest success rate by day eight in the Cytotec group, and this was a statistically significant finding (P = 0.02). 98% of women who were going to have an abortion regardless of whether they took one dosage of Cytotec or not, found that it was successful.

There was no discernible difference in the success rate of either therapy in relation to the gestational age of the patient.

Women who were given Cytotec had a significantly increased risk of experiencing a drop in hemoglobin of at least 3 g/dL (5% versus 1%, P=0.04).

Chapter 3: Dosage and Side Effects

Warnings

When determining whether or not to utilize a drug, it is important to consider the potential downsides of doing so with the potential benefits. When using this medication, the following things should be taken into consideration:

Allergies

Tell your doctor about any unusual or adverse reactions you may have had in the past to this drug or any other medicines you have taken. Inform your health care provider if you suffer from any additional forms of allergies, whether they be to foods, colours, preservatives, or animals, for example. When purchasing goods that do not require a prescription, it is important to carefully study the ingredient list on the label or container.

Pediatric

The association between age and the effects of misoprostol in the pediatric population has not been well investigated via the conduct of appropriate research.

Geriatric

In the proper tests that have been accomplished till this moment, geriatric-particular matters that might restrain the efficacy of misoprostol in older people have not been uncovered.

Breastfeeding

There have not been any appropriate tests performed on ladies to ascertain whether or not utilizing this medicine during nursing presents a damage to the child. Earlier than using any medication while breastfeeding, ensure that you have pondered the possible benefits versus the possible hazards.

Drug Interactions

In certain instances, it is OK to combine two distinct medications, even if there is a possibility that they would have an adverse interaction with one another. In certain circumstances, your physician may decide to adjust the dosage, or other preventative measures may be required. The following exchanges have been chosen because of the potential relevance they have; nonetheless, it should not be assumed that this list is exhaustive in any way.

The combination of this medication with any of the following medications may raise the risk of certain adverse effects; nevertheless, it is possible that taking both prescriptions together will provide the most beneficial therapy for you. If you are prescribed both medications at the same time, your physician may adjust the dosage or the frequency with which you take either one or both of the medications.

- Phenylbutazone

Different kinds of Interactions

Certain drugs should not be used while eating food, or just before or after eating specific kinds of food, since there is a potential that they will interact negatively with one another and cause harmful side effects. While taking some drugs, consuming alcohol or smoking could considerably enhance the probability of an interaction taking place. Talk to the medical professional who is treating you about whether or not it is safe to take your medicine with certain foods, beverages, or smoking.

Various Other Medical Concerns

It is possible that the usage of this medication will be impacted by the existence of other medical conditions. If you suffer from any other clinical issues, including but not limited to the following, be sure to inform your doctor:

- Dehydration
- Heart or circulatory system issues
- Inflammatory intestine disorder
- Stomach ulcerations

The Proper Dosage

Do not take more of this medication than your physician has told you to, do not take it more often than he or she specifies, and do not take it for a higher period than he or she specifies. All of these things are against the directives that your physician gave you. It is very necessary that you see your doctor before making any changes to the dose that was given to you or before stopping the usage of this medicine altogether.

This medication's package should contain a leaflet that provides information specific to the patient using it. In the absence of specific instructions from your doctor to the contrary, the best times to take misoprostol are either during or immediately after meals, followed by the last few hours before going to bed. Always use this drug on a full stomach to help minimize the chance of adverse reactions such as diarrhea, loose stools, and stomach cramps.

Precautions

Don't utilize this medicine if you are expecting or if you are trying to in the near future. If taken during pregnancy, this medication increases the risk of having an abortion, giving birth too soon, or having a child with a birth defect. Before you begin using this medication, you will need to have a pregnancy test that comes back negative within the last two weeks. After you stop taking this medication, you should not cease using your birth control method for at least one month.

You ought to begin using this medicine on the second or third day of your next menstruation, whichever comes first. Some individuals may experience nausea, stomach cramps, or diarrhea as a side effect of taking this medication. However, you should make an appointment with your primary care physician if the nausea, cramping, or diarrhea is severe or if it does not go away within a week. It's possible that the dose of misoprostol your doctor has prescribed for you will need to be decreased.

Side Effects

A drug may have some unintended side effects in addition to the results that are desired from taking it. Even while not all of these potential adverse effects may manifest themselves, if they do, you may require medical assistance.

Consult your physician as soon as possible if any of the following unwanted consequences manifest themselves:

Rare

- Cramps
- Heavy bleeding
- Painful menstruation

Unknown occurrence of the event

- Bladder pain bloody nose
- Stools that are bloody or dark and tarry
- Urine that is hazy or bloody
- Vision that is not clear
- Bodily pains or discomfort
- Chest pain
- Chills
- Confusion
- Constipation
- Cough
- Urination that is difficult, uncomfortable, or even scorching
- Having trouble breathing is a problem
- A challenge in terms of movement
- Swallowing is tough for the patient
- Dizziness
- A feeling similar to fainting, dizziness, or lightheadedness after rising too quickly from a seated or laying posture
- Congestion of the ears
- Shivering for no apparent reason
- Fever
- Frequent desire to urinate

- Headache
- Welts, itching, or a rash on the skin
- voice disappearing
- Discomfort in the lower back or the sides
- Muscular discomfort or stiffness
- Nasal congestion
- Nervousness
- Ache in the joints of the body
- Pale skin
- A throbbing sound in the ears
- A puffy or swollen appearance of the eyelids or the area surrounding the eyes, cheeks, lips, or tongue
- Runny nose
- Agonizing pains in the stomach
- Shivering
- A sluggish or rapid beating heart
- Sneezing
- Throat irritation
- Sweating
- Discomfort felt in the chest
- Respiratory issues brought on by physical activity
- Bruising or bleeding that is not normal
- Unexpected fatigue or a lack of strength

- Blood vomiting or the vomiting of something that looks like grounds for coffee

There is a possibility of experiencing some side effects, most of which do not normally require medical treatment. During therapy, when your body becomes used to the medication, these negative effects can disappear. In addition, the medical practitioner who is assisting you may be able to provide you with information regarding the avoidance or mitigation of certain of these adverse effects.

- Diarrhea
- Acid or sour stomach
- Belching
- Bloated
- Excess air or gas in the stomach or intestines
- Full feeling
- Heartburn
- Indigestion
- Passing gas
- Stomach discomfort or upset

Unknown occurrence of the event

- Pain in the breasts that may be accompanied by blistering, crusting, itching, or irritation of the skin

- Eyes that are burning, dry, or itching
- A continual ringing or buzzing or other inexplicable sounds in the ears
- A change in taste
- Skin that is cracked, dry, and scaled
- Symptoms such as sadness, frequent crying, hair loss or thinning, hearing loss, and hair loss can be caused by alopecia.
- A decrease in strength or a bereavement of vigor
- Pale pelt, blush, discomfort, or inflammation of the eye, lid, or the burden of the internal coating of the lid varies
- Loss of strength or a decrease in strength

Contraindications

Misoprostol is contraindicated:

- In women who are capable of bearing children but do not make use of methods of contraception that have been shown to be efficient.
- Due to the fact that misoprostol enhances uterine tenor and shrinkages in childbearing that can induce incomplete or entire eviction of the fruits of conception, it should be avoided in ladies who are expecting, in women whose childbearing has not been eliminated, or who are pro-

gramming a childbearing. It is not recommended to give misoprostol to a woman who is not pregnant or in whom pregnancy has not been ruled out until after taking the drug. There is a correlation between use during pregnancy and the occurrence of congenital defects in the offspring.

- Patients who have shown a severe sensitivity to miso-prostol, any other component of the product, or any other prostaglandins in the past.

Chapter 4: Clinical Uses

Peptic ulcers, also known as stomach ulcers or duodenal ulcers, are open sores that form on the stomach or upper small intestinal lining. These ulcers have the potential to spread throughout the gastrointestinal system. Peptic ulcers may arise from a number of different situations.

Stomach discomfort is the sign that a peptic ulcer is present the majority of the time.

Gastric ulcerations include:

- Ulcers of the stomach that grow on the inner coating of the belly.
- Ulcerations of the small intestine are weals that generate on the coating of the elevated section of the small bowel (duodenum).

Peptic ulcers are not the only type of bacterial infection that can produce ulcers in the digestive tract. Stress and the use of meals with a spicy flavor are not factors that lead to the development of peptic ulcers. Nonetheless, they have the capability to get the symptoms you are already experiencing worse.

Symptoms

- A painful churning in the stomach
- Intolerance to fatty meals characterized by a feeling of fullness, bloating, or belching
- Heartburn Nausea

Burning pain in the abdomen is one of the most typical signs of peptic ulcers. The annoyance is aggravated by belly sourness, as well as by a lack of nourishment in the stomach. Consuming specific meals that operate as a bumper against belly sourness or using a prescription that diminishes sourness productivity may often supply alleviation from the grief; nevertheless, the annoyance might come back. The majority of people who have peptic ulcers never ever experience any symptoms.

Ulcerations induce serious marks and manifestations far less regularly, yet they may involve the following:

- Expelling of belly substances or sap.
- Stools that are dark or pitchy, or bloody stools that are murky in color.
- Difficulty with breathing.
- Having a sensation of weakness.
- A nauseated stomach or puking.
- A decrease of weight for no evident motive.

- Adaptations of the appetite.

When need one to go to the physician?

You need to discuss with a care provider if you have any of the serious manifestations quoted above. If the pain subsides while using over-the-counter antacids or acid blockers but returns after you stop taking them, you should see your doctor.

Causes

Acid from the digestive system may devour the coating of the belly, generating a condition known as gastric ulceration disorder. Applying the acid might result in a painful open wound that may bleed.

The mucous lining of your digestive system protects the lining of your digestive tract from the acid in your stomach. However, if your stomach acid levels are too high or your mucus production is too low, you may get an ulcer.

Helicobacter pylori is a bacterium that is often encountered in the mucosa stratum that drapes and preserves the coatings that delimit the belly and bowel. Though the H. pylori bacterium often does not cause any problems, it has been linked to ulcer formation due to causing inflammation of the stomach's inner lining.

Utilization of certain analgesics on a consistent basis

It is possible for the lining of your stomach and small intestine to become irritated or inflamed if you regularly use aspirin or other nonsteroidal anti-inflammatory medicines (NSAIDs), which include some pain medications available over-the-counter and by prescription. These drugs include ibuprofen (sold under the brand names Advil and Motrin IB, among others), naproxen sodium (sold under the brand names Aleve and Anaprox DS, among others), and ketoprofen, among others. They don't comprehend acetaminophen in any form.

Determinants of Risk

You may have an elevated risk of peptic ulcers in addition to the hazards associated with using NSAIDs if any of the following apply to you:

Drink booze: The mucous lining of your stomach can get irritated and worn away by alcohol, and this can also lead to an increase in the quantity of stomach acid that is generated.

- Have stress that is not being handled.
- Eat dishes with a spicy kick.

Ulcers are not caused by these variables on their own, but they can make existing ulcers worse and make it harder for them to heal.

Complications

Peptic ulcers, if left untreated, can result in the generation of hemorrhagic conditions. It is possible for bleeding to cause a gradual loss of blood, which can result in anemia, or it can cause a significant loss of blood, which may require hospitalization or a blood transfusion. Vomit that is black or bloody, as well as feces that are black or bloody, might be the result of severe blood loss.

A hole, also known as a perforation, in the wall of your stomach, may put yourself at risk for a dangerous infection of your abdominal cavity if you have peptic ulcers because they can eat a hole through the wall of your stomach or small intestine.

Obstruction: Peptic ulcers can prevent food from moving through the digestive tract, which can lead to you feeling full more quickly, making you throw up, and causing you to lose weight either because of swelling caused by inflammation or because of scarring.

The number of prescriptions given for nonsteroidal anti-inflammatory drugs (NSAIDs) continues to rise, reaching over 22 million in the United Kingdom and over 70 million in the United

States annually. Due to the fact that aspirin and other NSAIDs are readily available as "over-the-counter" treatments, these data may not accurately reflect their true usage.

In the years to come, it is also reasonable to anticipate an increase in the consumption of these pharmaceuticals. This is due, in part, to the maturing of the population as a whole, and, in part, to the prospect of new and expanding indications for their use, most notably in the prevention of cancer and vascular disease. Because of this, it is essential to evaluate the safety of NSAIDs, as well as their potential adverse effects, and to think about how their safety may be enhanced. It has been known for a long time that nonsteroidal anti-inflammatory drugs can cause a variety of adverse effects, the most prevalent of which are digestive in nature.

This study will investigate the type, extent, and potential causes of the gastrointestinal side effects that are associated with the use of nonsteroidal anti-inflammatory drugs, as well as the potential means by which these effects might be mitigated or altered. Other side effects, including nephropathies, skin rashes, and hepatitis, have been linked to the use of NSAIDs; however, these complications are far less common than gastrointestinal issues.

Although specific data are difficult to get due to the difficulties of establishing proper control groups, endoscopic investigations have demonstrated this incidence. Patients who report gastrointestinal bleeding while using NSAIDs may have an equal incidence of gastric and duodenal ulceration. This is despite the fact that endoscopic investigations have a tendency to demonstrate more gastric than duodenal ulcers linked with NSAID usage. Dyspeptic symptoms can occur in as many as sixty percent of patients who take no steroidal anti-inflammatory drugs.

It has been calculated that the individual risk of being hospitalized due to gastrointestinal issues as a result of taking NSAIDs ranges anywhere from 1/50 to 1/150 patient-years. There is a one in one hundred to one in five hundred patient-years chance of an upper gastrointestinal hemorrhage, and there is a one in one thousand to one in five thousand patient-years chance of dying from something connected to the digestive system.

In addition to the stomach and duodenum, other regions of the gastrointestinal system, such as the esophagus, small intestine, and colon, have the potential to be harmed by the use of non-steroidal anti-inflammatory drugs.

There was no correlation between the patients' usage of NSAIDs and their deaths, according to the findings of a recent necropsy research that involved 713 individuals. Of those patients, 244 were prescribed NSAIDs in the six months before to their deaths, while the remaining 469 were not. It was discovered that 21.7% of patients taking NSAIDs had ulcers of the stomach or duodenum, compared to 12.3% of patients who were not taking NSAIDs (p0.001), and it was revealed that 8.4% of NSAID users had small intestinal ulceration, compared to 0.6% of patients who were not taking NSAIDs (p0.001). Enteroscopy has also shown that those who take NSAIDs are more likely to have damage to their small intestine. Patients who have suffered damage to their small intestine as a result of continuous use of NSAIDs may exhibit symptoms such as chronic iron deficiency anemia or hypoalbuminemia as a result of the loss of blood or protein. These patients may also exhibit overt bleeding, perforation, or strictures.

Chronic use of NSAIDs has been linked, albeit in extremely rare cases, to the development of oesophagitis, stricture formation, and ulceration in the oesophagus.

Smoking, an underlying respiratory or cardiovascular illness, and concurrent medication use—particularly corticosteroids, aspirin, and anticoagulants—are all considered to be among the highest risk factors. Utilization during surgery is another element that raises the risk. The nonsteroidal anti-inflammatory drugs azapropazone, ketoprofen, and piroxicam have the greatest individual risk, whereas ibuprofen, diclofenac, and etodolac pose the lowest individual risk. In addition to using more than one NSAID, a greater risk is related with higher dosages of the medication. Aspirin used at relatively modest doses for preventative purposes, which is common practice in today's world, is associated with an increased risk of gastrointestinal problems. The possibility of an interaction between NSAIDs and an increased risk of ulceration caused by Helicobacter pylori is the subject of some controversy, and this topic will be covered in a later section. The weight of evidence from clinical studies and the physiological associations between the two seems to support the hypothesis that there is some interaction taking place, particularly in those patients who are at a high risk and maybe in those who have bled.

Why do NSAIDs induce gastrointestinal damage?

The cyclooxygenase (COX) mechanisms that lead to the formation of prostanoids are disrupted by nonsteroidal anti-inflammatory drugs (prostaglandins, prostacyclin, and thromboxane). This reduces the efficiency of the mucus-bicarbonate barrier, which in turn makes it more likely that stomach acid and probably also pepsin would cause harm. This reduces the mucosal protection afforded by the mucosa. It's possible that the fact that most NSAIDs are also weak acids is another factor that contributes to the problem.

It is now common knowledge that COX may be found in two distinct isoforms: COX-1 and COX-2. The expression and regulation of these two isoforms in various tissues is quite different from one another.

It also has a role in the preservation of vascular homoeostasis and excellent renal function, in addition to playing a role in the maintenance of normal physiological processes in a large number of other cell types. This is a crucial "housekeeping" function to fulfill. It would appear that platelets solely contain COX-1. Gastric ulcerations are open weals that grow on the internal coating of your belly and the elevated segment of your small bowel. Peptic ulcers are a painful condition that has the ability to propagate to other places of the organism. There are multiple definite elements that have been connected to the development of ulcers in the peptic tract. Patients will almost always experience pain in the stomach when a peptic ulcer is present since this is where the ulcer is located.

Peptic ulcers include:

Ulcerations of the belly are open weals that grow on the coating of the belly, and they are sometimes very painful. Duodenal ulcers are open lesions that grow on the coating of the upper region of the small bowel and are recognized as peptic ulcerations. Ulcers of the duodenum may be caused by many diverse aspects.

Both a contagion with the microorganism Helicobacter pylori (H. pylori) and the utilization of pain-relieving medications for a lengthy period of time are the most frequent sources of gastric ulcerations. Gastric ulcerations are aching lesions that form in the coating of the belly and duodenum. Ulcers in the digestive system may be caused by more than only peptic ulcer disease; other types of bacterial infections can have the same effect. Peptic ulcers are not caused by anxiety or the consumption of foods with a spicy taste since these are not variables that contribute to their development. However, there is a possibility that they will make the symptoms that you are currently experiencing much more severe.

Some of the symptoms include an uncomfortable churning in the stomach, inability to tolerate fatty meals, sometimes accompanied by uncomfortable sensations such as bloating, fullness, and burping

Burning in the belly and Nausea

Burning pain in the belly is one of the most prevalent symptoms associated with peptic ulcers. Peptic ulcers are defined by a variety of different symptoms. The pain is exacerbated not only by the acid that is present in the stomach, but also by the fact that there is no food present in the stomach at this time. Eating certain meals that act as a buffer against stomach acid or taking a prescription that suppresses the formation of acid are both common ways to ease the pain associated with heartburn and peptic ulcers. However, even if relief is found, it is possible that the pain may eventually return. There is a possibility that the discomfort will be more severe in the middle of the night or during the hours that pass between meals.

The great majority of people, who have peptic ulcers never, ever report any symptoms of the ailment, even though it is quite likely that they have it. Ulcers produce significant signs and symptoms far less often, but when they do, they might include the following:

- Expulsion of stomach contents or blood, which may or may not be colored, black or tarry stools, or bloody stools that are dark in color.
- Expulsion of the contents of the stomach or blood, which may or may not have a crimson or black tint to it.
- Problems with one's capacity to breathe; experiencing a sensation comparable to that of fainting; having a stomach full of nausea or vomiting up; experiencing a loss of weight for which there is no clear cause; experiencing dizziness or lightheadedness; alterations that take place in one's hunger and satiety levels.

When is the most pertinent time to visit a health care provider?

If you are experiencing any of the significant signs or symptoms that have been mentioned in the previous paragraphs, you need to schedule an appointment with a qualified medical practitioner as soon as you can. If the pain is relieved by over-the-counter antacids and acid blockers but then returns after treatment, you should schedule an appointment with your primary care physician as soon as possible.

Causes

Gastric ulcerations may develop when the sourness in the gastrointestinal system devours the internal side of the belly or the small bowel, which can result in the development of peptic ulcers. This acid eats away at the inner surface, which may lead to the development of peptic ulcers. Once the acid has been applied, it may cause a painful open wound that is prone to bleeding. This wound can occur after the acid has been delivered.

The mucous layer that is ordinarily present in your digestive system serves as a barrier between that layer and the acid that is found in your stomach. Your digestive system is shielded from the acid that is produced in your stomach by this layer. Nevertheless, you run the risk of developing an ulceration if the quantity of sourness in your belly is raised or if the quantity of mucus in your belly is decreased. Both of these things might cause your stomach to produce less mucus and more acid. Both of these factors might result in your stomach producing less mucus and more acid than usual.

The subsequent reasons are among the most often offered:

The mucosa stratum that drapes and preserves the coatings that delimit the belly and small bowel is a frequent home for the bacteria that generate helicobacter pylori infection. This layer also acts as an obstruction between the belly and the small bowel. In most cases, the H. pylori bacteria do not cause any difficulties; nevertheless, it may induce inflammation of the inner layer of the stomach, which can lead to the creation of an ulcer. In most cases, the bacteria do not give rise to any issues.

It is not completely comprehensible how illnesses brought on by H. pylori may be transmitted from one man to another. It is possible for it to spread from one person to another via the act of kissing or through other types of intimate physical contact. H. pylori is an illness that may possibly develop in a person if they consume contaminated food or water. This infection can be propagated from subject to subject.

Constant use of certain analgesics

If you utilize aspirin or any other pain-relieving medications con-sistently, the coating of your belly and small bowel can get dis-pleased. This is one of the possible adverse reactions of these medications. Among these drugs are several pain relievers that are available without a doctor's prescription or that may be ac-quired over the counter.

There are many different categories of drugs. In addition to non-steroidal anti-inflammatory medicines, often known as NSAIDs, the use of certain additional medications, including steroids, anti-coagulants, low-dose aspirin, selective serotonin reuptake inhibi-tors, also known as SSRIs, alendronate (Fosamax), and risedronate (Actonel), may considerably increase the likelihood of developing ulcers.

Chapter 5: Frequently Asked Questions

1) Can I get Cytotec without a prescription?

This drug may only be procured with a medical recipe from your doctor.

2) Can Cytotec pills cause infertility?

Although there is no proven connection between taking an abortion pill and infertility, there is evidence that doing so increases the risk of difficulties with a subsequent pregnancy.

A research on abortion that was carried out in Denmark looked at the effects of having one on a woman's ability to have children in the future. The research looked at data from 12,000 different women who had abortions during the years of 1999 and 2004.

They investigated the likelihood of ectopic or tubal pregnancies, which occur when a fertilized egg implants itself in a location other than the uterus, among women who had had both surgical and medicinal procedures to terminate a pregnancy.

The researchers found that tubal pregnancies occurred at the same rate – approximately 2.5% of the time – in both surgical and medical abortions. While the study did not identify any additional side effects on fertility, they did find that tubal pregnancies occurred in both.

3) Is Cytotec an abortion pill?

It is true that this medication will prevent the pregnancy from progressing.

4) Is Cytotec safe for abortion?

This oral contraceptive pill is exceedingly dependable, and there are no known risks associated with its use. It is estimated that millions of women have been able to terminate their pregnancies with this technique, making it one of the most common forms of abortion.

Because of this, there is no hazard to your next childbearing or to your overall well-being, unless there is a problem that is very rare and significant that is not addressed. Except for that, there is no risk at all. There is no correlation between having an abortion and an increased risk of breast cancer or a reduction in fertility. Having a termination of pregnancy does not influence a person's ability to have more children.

It does not put a woman at risk for difficulties in subsequent pregnancies, such as birth defects, premature delivery or low birth weight, ectopic pregnancy, miscarriage, or the death of a child and it does not increase the likelihood of a woman having an abortion.

After an abortion, a person is statistically approximately as likely to experience serious mental issues in the long run as they are after giving birth. People who are forced to terminate a pregnancy due to health concerns, people who do not have support surrounding their decision to have an abortion, and people who have a history of mental health issues are more likely to experience these types of complications after the procedure. After having an abortion, the majority of people report feeling relieved.

5) Can Cytotec alone cause an abortion?

Women who are seeking an abortion in the first trimester of their pregnancy have a fair alternative in the form of misoprostol alone because it is both effective and safe.

6) After taking a Cytotec pill, how many days will I bleed?

You need to be aware of when the cramps and bleeding are expected to begin, as well as what issues to look out for. You need to also obviously realize that everybody is diverse, and that there is no specific time frame in which you should lose blood, or quantify the amount of blood you should observe. This is a matter that you absolutely need to understand. When you take misoprostol, it is normal for the bleeding to be thicker than usual, and it is also common that there are blood clots. On the other hand, if an abortion is performed at a very early stage of your pregnancy, there is a possibility that there will be no clots. It is possible for bleeding to begin anywhere between 24 and 72 hours after taking misoprostol.

If it hasn't started by the time the 72-hour mark has passed or if the bleeding is mild, this indicates that the abortion did not take place successfully. Within the first 24 hours after using miso-prostol, most women experience the most bleeding, which typically peaks between 2 and 5 hours after taking the medication and then gradually decreases. After the tissue has been evacuated, the cramping, which is another significant adverse consequence of medical abortion, should begin to improve.

After having a medical abortion, most women bleed for between 9 and 14 days, however it is not unheard for some women to bleed for as long as four weeks. It is also possible for the bleeding to cease completely after it has been extremely severe for a few days, or it may stop intermittently. Alternately, bleeding that is similar to a period might continue for several weeks after the period has ended. After using the termination pill, your womb will begin to empty itself. Since it is essential that your uterus empty itself entirely, it is OK for this process to take some time.

7) Can Cytotec affect a 2-month pregnancy?

It is only possible to have a termination up to 24 weeks into a pregnancy, both medical and surgical.

At the first 24 weeks of pregnancy, it is only possible to have an abortion in very particular circumstances, such as when the mother's life is in danger or when there are concerns with the baby's development. Abortions are not permitted after this point in the pregnancy.

8) .Is Cytotec a prohibited drug?

No, it's not. Misoprostol has a cheaper price point, a longer shelf life, and does not need to be refrigerated in comparison to other synthetic prostaglandin analogues. In addition to this, it is easily accessible in any territory of the world.

9) What stage of pregnancy can Cytotec work effectively?

It has been proved that the combination of misoprostol and mifepristone can successfully induce a medical abortion up to 9 weeks into a pregnancy. The rate of effective complete abortions declined to less than sixty percent when used alone. This is the first randomized research to compare the efficacy of taking misoprostol with water to taking misoprostol by itself for inducing a medical abortion in the first trimester of pregnancy in women who were less than 9 weeks pregnant.

A total of eighty women were split into two groups, group 1 receiving misoprostol mixed with water, and group 2 receiving the placebo (misoprostol alone). Misoprostol in a dose of 800 micrograms was administered vaginally on days 1, 3, and 5. Complete abortion was determined to have occurred if the woman who underwent medical abortion did not require any vacuum aspiration during the time leading up to the return of her first menstrual period after the abortion. A standardized questionnaire was used both during and after the abortion to gather data on the frequency of adverse effects and evaluate the acceptability of the procedure. It appeared that the total abortion rate was greater when water was introduced. In all groups, gastrointestinal adverse effects occurred frequently but were generally well tolerated. Because of the high incidence of failure, an overall forty percent of the women said they would choose surgery as their technique of choice in the future. Even though adding water helps enhance the results, this approach is probably not one that can be used in clinical settings because it has an overall rate of complete abortion that is 85 percent. We have come to the conclusion that adding water to misoprostol pills does not increase the medication's effectiveness when used for medical abortion in the first trimester. Due to the high failure rate and low acceptance, Cytotec alone is not advised for use in clinical abortions (up to 10 weeks of childbearing).

10) What are other remedies for abortion except for Cytotec?

When several supplements are ingested in significant quantities, or mixed into infusions, they are said to have the potential to act as abortive.

Vitamin C, parsley, Dong Quai, rose hips, ginger root, chamomile, and black cohosh were all utilized by around half of the participants in one study that was conducted in 2021 and cited as a Trusted Source. Others relied on painkillers, antibiotics, birth control pills, and caffeine tablets to get through the ordeal.

None of these drugs have been evaluated or endorsed for use in the induction of an abortion, and several of them, even in trace doses, have the potential to cause significant damage.

Printed by
Youcanprint